BLOOD SUGAR DIET SOLUTION

Practical Tips for Stability and Wellness

Emily J. Headley

Emily J. Headley

TABLE OF CONTENTS

INTRODUCTION

Welcome to "Blood Sugar Diet Solution." In the pages of this book, we embark on a journey to demystify the complexities surrounding blood sugar management and provide you with practical solutions to support your health and well-being. Whether you're seeking to prevent diabetes, manage existing conditions, or simply adopt a healthier lifestyle, the insights and strategies shared here will empower you to take control of your blood sugar levels and improve your overall quality of life.

Understanding blood sugar and its impact on our health is crucial in today's world, where conditions like diabetes and insulin resistance are increasingly prevalent. But the topic can often seem overwhelming, filled with confusing terminology and conflicting advice. That's why our approach in this book is straightforward and accessible, aimed at providing you with the knowledge and tools you need to make informed decisions about your health.

Throughout these pages, we'll cover everything from the basics of blood sugar regulation to practical tips for incorporating healthy habits into your daily routine. You'll learn how factors such as diet, exercise, stress management, and sleep can all influence your blood sugar levels, and how making simple changes in these areas can have a profound impact on your health.

But before we dive into the specifics, let's take a moment to understand what blood sugar is and why it's so important to keep it in balance.

At its core, blood sugar, also known as glucose, is the primary source of energy for our bodies. It comes from the foods we eat, particularly those rich in carbohydrates, which are broken down into glucose during digestion and released into the bloodstream. From there, glucose is transported to our cells, where it's used to fuel various physiological processes, from powering our muscles during exercise to fueling our brain for cognitive function.

However, maintaining the right balance of blood sugar is crucial. Too much glucose in the bloodstream can lead to hyperglycemia, a condition associated with diabetes and other health complications. On the other hand, chronically low blood sugar levels, known as hypoglycemia, can also have serious consequences, including dizziness, weakness, and even loss of consciousness.

The body has an intricate system in place to regulate blood sugar levels, primarily through the actions of insulin, a hormone produced by the pancreas. When blood sugar levels rise after a meal, insulin is released to help transport glucose from the bloodstream into the cells, where it's either used for immediate energy or stored for later use. When blood sugar levels drop, another hormone called glucagon signals the liver to release stored glucose into the bloodstream to maintain a stable supply of energy.

However, this delicate balance can be disrupted by various factors, including poor dietary choices, lack of physical activity, stress, and inadequate sleep. Over time, these factors can contribute to insulin resistance, a condition in which the body's cells become less responsive to insulin's actions, leading to elevated blood sugar levels and an elevated danger of diabetes.

But the good news is that many of these risk factors are modifiable through lifestyle changes. By adopting a balanced diet, engaging in regular physical activity, managing stress effectively, and prioritizing sleep, you can significantly improve your blood sugar control and reduce your risk of developing diabetes and other related conditions.

Throughout this book, we'll explore these topics in more detail, providing you with evidence-based recommendations and practical strategies for implementing healthy habits into your daily life. Whether you're looking to lose weight, improve your energy levels, or simply feel better overall, the principles of blood sugar management can serve as a foundation for achieving your health and wellness goals.

So, if you're ready to take control of your blood sugar and embark on a journey towards better health, I invite you to join me as we explore the "Blood Sugar Diet Solution" together. Whether you're a beginner looking for guidance or someone who's already well-versed in the topic, there's something here for everyone. Let's empower ourselves with knowledge and take the first step towards a healthier, happier future.

CHAPTER ONE:

THE BASICS OF BLOOD SUGAR

In this chapter, we'll delve into the fundamentals of blood sugar, exploring what it is, the crucial role of insulin, and how to understand blood sugar levels. By grasping these essential concepts, you'll lay the foundation for effective blood sugar management and pave the way toward better health and vitality.

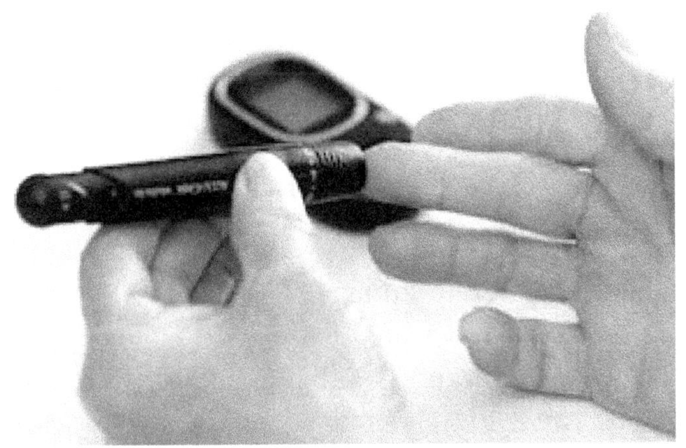

What is Blood Sugar?

Blood sugar, also known as glucose, serves as the primary source of energy for our bodies. It's derived from the foods we eat, particularly carbohydrates, which are broken down during digestion into glucose molecules. Once absorbed into the bloodstream, glucose is transported to cells throughout the body, providing fuel for various physiological processes, including cellular metabolism, muscle contraction, and brain function.

Maintaining blood sugar within a narrow range is essential for optimal health. Too much or too little glucose in the blood can have detrimental effects on our well-being. When blood sugar levels are too high, as in the case of diabetes, it can lead to complications such as cardiovascular disease, kidney damage, and nerve damage. Conversely, low blood sugar levels, known as hypoglycemia, can cause symptoms like dizziness, fatigue, and confusion, and if severe, can lead to unconsciousness or seizures.

The Role of Insulin

Insulin plays a very important part in regulating blood sugar levels. Produced by the pancreas, insulin acts as a key that unlocks cells, allowing glucose to enter and be utilized for energy. When blood sugar levels rise after a meal, the pancreas releases insulin into the bloodstream to facilitate the uptake of glucose by cells, thereby lowering blood sugar levels.

In addition to promoting glucose uptake, insulin also helps store excess glucose in the liver and muscles in the form of glycogen for later use. This ensures a steady supply of energy between meals and during periods of increased physical activity.

In individuals with diabetes, the production or action of insulin is impaired, leading to abnormal blood sugar levels. In type 1 diabetes, the pancreas fails to produce insulin due to the autoimmune destruction of insulin-producing beta cells. In type 2 diabetes, the body becomes resistant to the effects of insulin or doesn't produce enough insulin to meet its needs. Proper management of diabetes involves maintaining blood sugar levels within a target range through a combination of medication, diet, exercise, and lifestyle modifications.

Understanding Blood Sugar Levels

Blood sugar levels are measured in milligrams of glucose per deciliter of blood (mg/dL) and can fluctuate throughout the day in response to various factors such as food intake, physical activity, stress, and medication. Normal fasting blood sugar levels typically range between 70 to 100 mg/dL, while postprandial (after-meal) blood sugar levels may rise temporarily but should return to within the normal range within a few hours.

Continuous monitoring of blood sugar levels is essential for individuals with diabetes to prevent complications and optimize health outcomes. This can be achieved through self-monitoring using a blood glucose meter or continuous glucose monitoring (CGM) devices, which provide real-time data on blood sugar levels and trends.

Interpreting blood sugar readings involves understanding target ranges and patterns over time. Consistently high or low blood sugar levels may indicate the need for adjustments to medication, diet, or lifestyle factors. Keeping a blood sugar log and working closely with healthcare providers can help individuals with diabetes make informed decisions about managing their condition effectively.

By gaining a solid understanding of blood sugar basics, including what it is, the role of insulin, and how to interpret blood sugar levels, you'll be better equipped to navigate the complexities of blood sugar management and take proactive steps toward achieving optimal health and well-being. In the following chapters, we'll explore strategies for maintaining blood sugar balance through diet, exercise, stress management, and other lifestyle interventions. With knowledge and dedication, you can empower yourself to take control of your blood sugar and live a healthier, more vibrant life.

CHAPTER TWO:
ASSESSING YOUR CURRENT HEALTH

In this chapter, we'll explore essential methods for assessing your current health about blood sugar levels. Understanding how and when to test your blood sugar, interpreting the results, and identifying risk factors for blood sugar imbalance are crucial steps in taking control of your health and well-being.

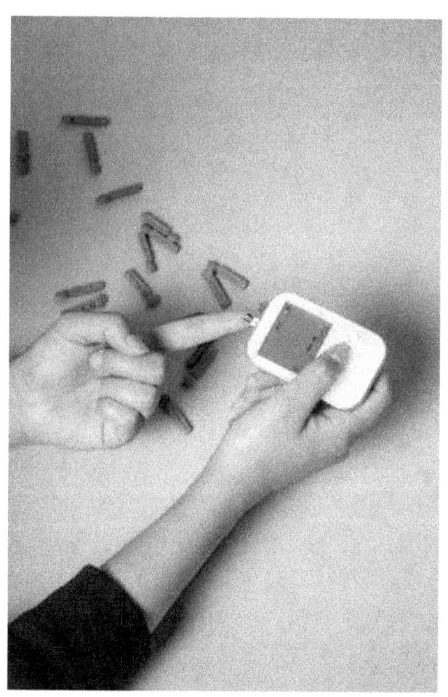

Blood Sugar Testing: How, When, and Why

Blood sugar testing is a simple yet valuable tool for monitoring your health and managing blood sugar levels effectively. Testing your blood sugar involves measuring the concentration of glucose in your bloodstream at a specific moment in time. This can be done using a handheld blood glucose meter, which requires a small drop of blood obtained by pricking your finger with a lancet.

How to Test: To perform a blood sugar test, wash your hands with soap and water and dry them thoroughly. Use the lancet device to prick the side of your fingertip and collect a small drop of blood. Place the blood onto a test strip inserted into the meter and wait for the result to appear on the meter's display.

When to Test: The frequency of blood sugar testing may vary depending on individual circumstances, such as the type of diabetes, medication regimen, and overall health status. Common times for testing include before meals, after meals, before bedtime, and during periods of physical activity or illness.

Why Test: Regular blood sugar testing allows you to track your progress, identify patterns, and make informed decisions about managing your blood sugar levels. It provides valuable insight into how your body responds to food, medication, exercise, and other factors that influence blood sugar.

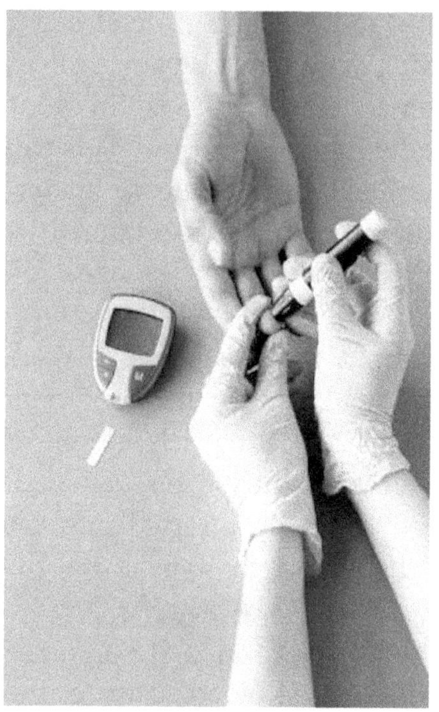

Interpreting Blood Sugar Readings

Interpreting blood sugar readings involves understanding the significance of your test results and how they relate to your overall health. Blood sugar levels are typically measured in milligrams of glucose per deciliter of blood (mg/dL) and can vary throughout the day. Here are some general guidelines for interpreting blood sugar readings:

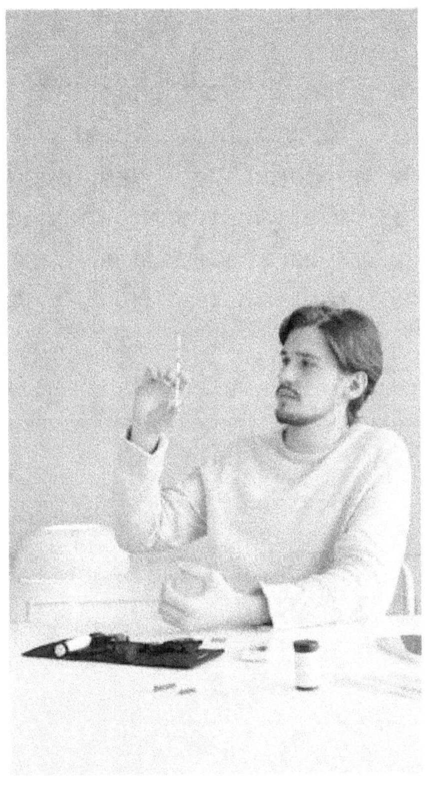

Normal Range: Fasting blood sugar levels between 70 to 100 mg/dL are considered normal for most individuals. Postprandial (after-meal) blood sugar levels may rise temporarily but should return to within the normal range within a few hours.

High Blood Sugar (Hyperglycemia): Blood sugar levels consistently above 180 mg/dL may indicate hyperglycemia, a condition commonly associated with diabetes. Symptoms of hyperglycemia include increased thirst, frequent urination, fatigue, and blurred vision.

Low Blood Sugar (Hypoglycemia): Blood sugar levels below 70 mg/dL may indicate hypoglycemia, a condition characterized by abnormally low blood sugar levels. Symptoms of hypoglycemia include shakiness, sweating, dizziness, confusion, and hunger.

Identifying Risk Factors for Blood Sugar Imbalance

Several factors can increase your risk of developing blood sugar imbalances, including:
Family History: A family history of diabetes or other metabolic disorders can increase your risk of developing blood sugar imbalances.

Obesity or Overweight: Being overweight or obese can impair insulin sensitivity and increase the risk of insulin resistance and type 2 diabetes.

Unhealthy Diet: Diets high in refined carbohydrates, added sugars, and processed foods can contribute to blood sugar imbalances and insulin resistance.

Physical Inactivity: Lack of regular physical activity can impair glucose metabolism and increase the risk of insulin resistance and type 2 diabetes.

Stress: Chronic stress can elevate blood sugar levels through the release of stress hormones like cortisol, contributing to insulin resistance and metabolic dysfunction.
By identifying these risk factors and addressing them proactively, you can reduce your risk of developing blood sugar imbalances and improve your overall health and well-being.

Lastly, assessing your current health about blood sugar levels involves regular testing, interpreting the results accurately, and identifying risk factors for blood sugar imbalance. By taking proactive steps to monitor and manage your blood sugar levels, you can optimize your health and reduce your risk of developing diabetes and other metabolic disorders. In the following chapters, we'll explore strategies for maintaining blood sugar balance through diet, exercise, stress management, and other lifestyle interventions.

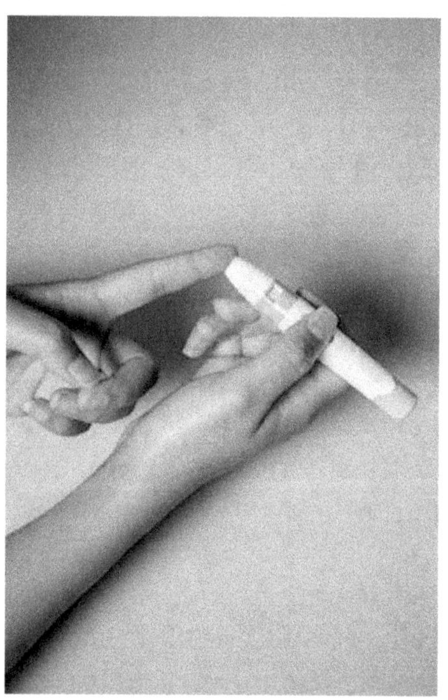

CHAPTER THREE:
THE IMPACT OF DIET ON BLOOD SUGAR

In this chapter, we'll delve into the profound influence of diet on blood sugar levels. Understanding the role of carbohydrates, the significance of the glycemic index and glycemic load, and the contribution of protein and fat to blood sugar regulation is essential for making informed choices in the diet that promote optimum health and quality of life.

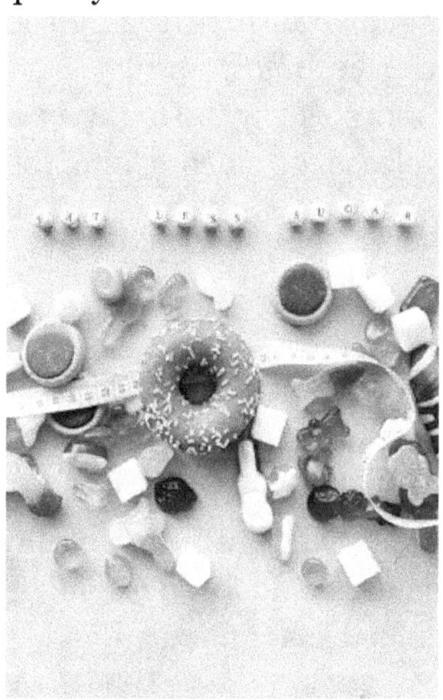

Carbohydrates: Friend or Foe?

Carbohydrates are a primary source of energy for the body, providing glucose that fuels cellular processes and activities. However, not all carbohydrates are created equal, and their impact on blood sugar levels can vary widely depending on their composition and how they're processed.

Simple carbohydrates, such as those found in refined grains, sugary snacks, and sweetened beverages, are quickly digested and absorbed into the bloodstream, causing a rapid spike in blood sugar levels. On the other hand, complex carbohydrates, such as those found in whole grains, legumes, fruits, and vegetables, are digested more slowly, resulting in a gradual and sustained release of glucose into the bloodstream.

In my own experience, I've found that opting for whole, unprocessed carbohydrates, such as brown rice, quinoa, and sweet potatoes, helps me maintain stable blood sugar levels throughout the day. By prioritizing nutrient-dense, fiber-rich foods over sugary treats and refined snacks, I've been able to better manage my energy levels and avoid the highs and lows associated with blood sugar fluctuations.

The Glycemic Index and Glycemic Load

The glycemic index (GI) is a measure of how quickly a carbohydrate-containing food raises blood sugar levels compared to pure glucose. Foods with a high GI are rapidly digested and absorbed, causing a sharp increase in blood sugar levels, whole foods with a low GI are digested more slowly, gradually increasing blood sugar levels.

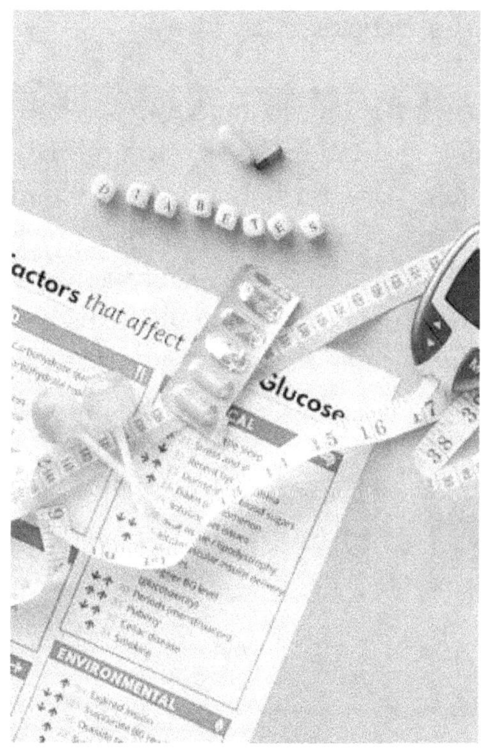

In addition to the GI, the glycemic load (GL) takes into account both the quality and quantity of carbohydrates in a serving of food. It provides a more accurate assessment of a food's impact on blood sugar levels by considering the portion size as well as the GI.

For example, watermelon has a high GI but a low GL because it contains relatively few carbohydrates per serving. On the other hand, white bread has a high GI and a high GL because it contains a larger amount of carbohydrates per serving.

By choosing foods with a low to moderate GI and GL, such as whole grains, legumes, non-starchy vegetables, and fruits, you can help stabilize blood sugar levels and reduce the risk of insulin resistance and type 2 diabetes. Incorporating a variety of foods with different GI and GL values into your meals can further enhance blood sugar control and promote overall health.

Protein and Fat: Their Role in Blood Sugar Regulation

While carbohydrates have the most significant impact on blood sugar levels, protein and fat also play important roles in blood sugar regulation. Unlike carbohydrates, protein and fat have minimal direct effects on blood sugar levels and are metabolized more slowly, providing a steady source of energy over time.

Protein-rich foods, such as lean meats, poultry, fish, eggs, tofu, and legumes, can help stabilize blood sugar levels by slowing down the absorption of carbohydrates and promoting satiety. Including protein with each meal and snack can help prevent spikes and crashes in blood sugar levels and support weight management goals.

Similarly, dietary fat, found in foods like avocados, nuts, seeds, olive oil, and fatty fish, can help slow down the absorption of carbohydrates and promote feelings of fullness and satisfaction. Incorporating healthy fats into your meals can help improve blood sugar control and reduce cravings for sugary foods.

In my dietary journey, I've found that balancing carbohydrates with protein and fat helps me maintain stable blood sugar levels and avoid the energy crashes that often accompany high-carbohydrate meals. By focusing on whole, nutrient-dense foods and incorporating a variety of macronutrients into my diet, I've been able to achieve better blood sugar control and overall well-being.

In conclusion, the impact of diet on blood sugar levels is profound and multifaceted. By choosing whole, unprocessed carbohydrates, paying attention to the glycemic index and glycemic load of foods, and balancing carbohydrates with protein and fat, you can support optimal blood sugar control and promote long-term health and vitality. In the following chapters, we'll explore practical strategies for designing a blood sugar-friendly diet plan and implementing it into your daily life.

CHAPTER FOUR: DESIGNING YOUR BLOOD SUGAR DIET PLAN

In this chapter, we'll outline the essential steps for creating a blood sugar-friendly diet plan that supports optimal blood sugar control and promotes overall health and well-being. From setting goals for blood sugar control to crafting balanced meal plans and providing sample meal ideas and recipes, you'll learn practical strategies for designing a diet plan that works for you.

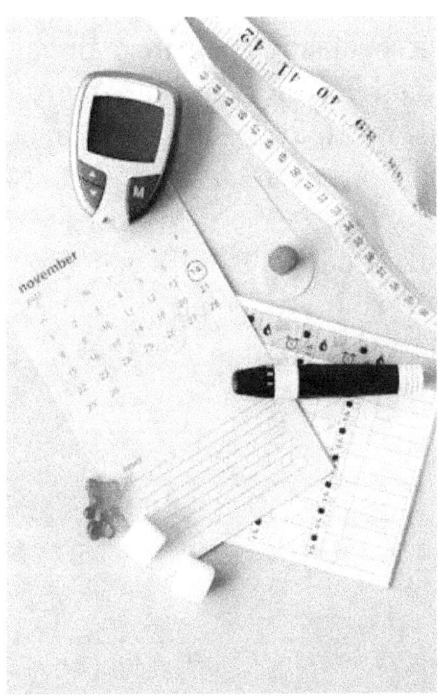

Setting Goals for Blood Sugar Control

Setting clear and achievable goals is the first step in designing an effective blood sugar diet plan. Whether you're looking to lower your fasting blood sugar levels, improve postprandial glucose response, or enhance overall glycemic control, defining specific, measurable, and realistic goals is key to success.

For example, a goal might be to reduce fasting blood sugar levels from 120 mg/dL to 100 mg/dL within three months by making dietary and lifestyle modifications. Another goal might be to maintain postprandial blood sugar levels below 140 mg/dL two hours after meals by choosing lower-glycemic foods and practicing portion control.

By identifying your individual goals for blood sugar control, you can tailor your diet plan to address specific needs and track your progress over time.

Creating a Balanced Meal Plan

A balanced meal plan is essential for managing blood sugar levels and promoting overall health. Aim to include a variety of nutrient-dense foods from all food groups, including carbohydrates, protein, healthy fats, fruits, vegetables, and fiber-rich foods.

Carbohydrates: Choose complex carbohydrates with a low to moderate glycemic index, such as whole grains, legumes, non-starchy vegetables, and fruits. Limit simple carbohydrates and refined sugars, such as sugary snacks, desserts, and processed foods.

Protein: Include lean sources of protein with each meal and snack, such as poultry, fish, eggs, tofu, legumes, and low-fat dairy products. Protein helps stabilize blood sugar levels and promotes feelings of fullness and satisfaction.

Healthy Fats: Incorporate sources of healthy fats into your diet, such as avocados, nuts, seeds, olive oil, and fatty fish. Healthy fats provide essential nutrients and help slow down the absorption of carbohydrates, promoting stable blood sugar levels.

Fiber: Choose fiber-rich foods, such as whole grains, fruits, vegetables, legumes, and nuts, which help regulate blood sugar levels, improve satiety, and support digestive health.

Sample Meal Plans and Recipes

To help you get started with your blood sugar diet plan, here are two sample meal plans and recipes that demonstrate how to create balanced meals that support optimal blood sugar control:

Sample Meal Plan 1:

Breakfast: Greek yogurt with berries, almonds, and chia seeds
Snack: Carrot sticks with hummus
Lunch: Quinoa salad with mixed vegetables, grilled chicken, and avocado
Snack: Apple slices with almond butter

Sample Meal Plan 2:

Breakfast: Oatmeal topped with sliced banana, walnuts, and cinnamon
Snack: Celery sticks with peanut butter
Lunch: Spinach salad with grilled shrimp, cherry tomatoes, feta cheese, and balsamic vinaigrette
Snack: Greek yogurt with sliced strawberries

These sample meal plans provide a framework for building balanced meals that promote stable blood sugar levels and support overall health. Feel free to customize them according to your preferences and dietary needs.

Finally, designing a blood sugar diet plan involves setting goals for blood sugar control, creating a balanced meal plan, and incorporating nutrient-dense foods that support optimal blood sugar regulation. By following these practical strategies and incorporating sample meal ideas and recipes into your daily routine, you can take control of your blood sugar levels and achieve better health and well-being. In the following chapters, we'll explore additional strategies for maintaining blood sugar balance through exercise, stress management, and other lifestyle interventions.

CHAPTER FIVE: LIFESTYLE STRATEGIES FOR BLOOD SUGAR MANAGEMENT

In this chapter, we'll explore lifestyle strategies that play a crucial role in blood sugar management. From incorporating regular exercise and physical activity to implementing stress management techniques and prioritizing quality sleep, these lifestyle interventions can significantly impact blood sugar levels and overall health.

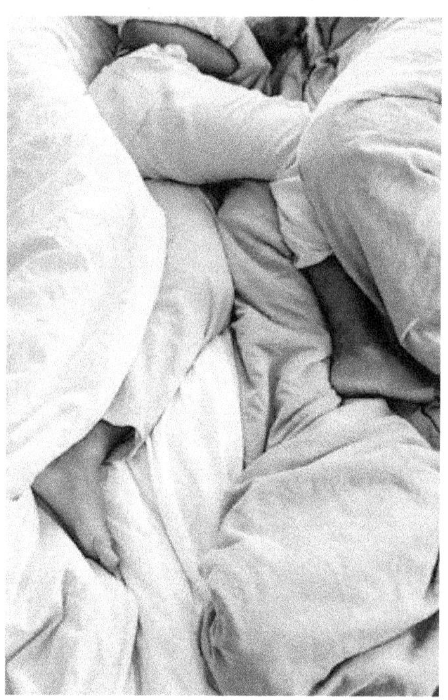

Exercise and Physical Activity Recommendations

Regular exercise and physical activity are essential components of a healthy lifestyle and play a key role in blood sugar management. Exercise helps improve insulin sensitivity, allowing cells to better absorb glucose from the bloodstream and utilize it for energy. It also promotes weight loss, reduces inflammation, and enhances cardiovascular health.

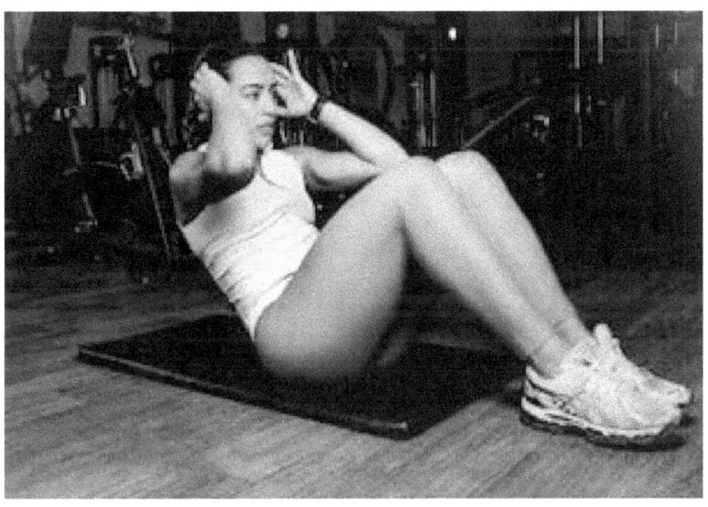

Examples of exercise and physical activity that can benefit blood sugar management include:

Aerobic Exercise: Activities such as walking, jogging, cycling, swimming, and dancing can help lower blood sugar levels and improve insulin sensitivity.

Strength Training: Resistance exercises, such as weightlifting, bodyweight exercises, and resistance band workouts, can increase muscle mass and improve glucose metabolism.

Flexibility and Balance Exercises: Yoga, tai chi, and Pilates can help reduce stress, improve flexibility, and promote overall well-being.

To engage in at least 150 minutes of moderate to vigorous intensity aerobic exercise or 75 minutes of high-intensity aerobic exercise per week, along with two or more days of strength training targeting major muscle groups.

Stress Management Techniques

Chronic stress can have detrimental effects on blood sugar levels and overall health. When we're stressed, the body releases stress hormones like cortisol and adrenaline, which can cause blood sugar levels to rise and promote insulin resistance over time.

To manage stress effectively and support blood sugar management, consider incorporating stress management techniques into your daily routine:

Deep Breathing: Practice deep breathing exercises to promote relaxation and reduce stress levels. Slowly and deeply breathe, inhaling through your nose as well as out of your mouth.

Mindfulness meditation: to cultivate awareness of the present moment and reduce stress, engage in mindful meditation. Focus on your breath, sensations in your body, or sounds in your environment.

Yoga and Tai Chi: Participate in yoga or tai chi classes to promote relaxation, reduce muscle tension, and improve overall well-being.

Hobbies and Leisure Activities: Engage in hobbies and activities that bring you joy and relaxation, such as gardening, painting, reading, or spending time in nature.

By incorporating stress management techniques into your daily routine, you can reduce the impact of stress on blood sugar levels and promote overall health and well-being.

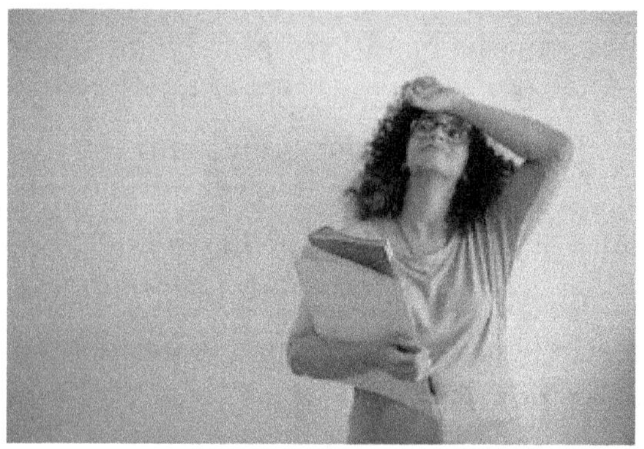

The Importance of Quality Sleep

Quality sleep is essential for maintaining optimal blood sugar levels and overall health. Poor sleep habits, such as irregular sleep patterns, insufficient sleep duration, and disrupted sleep quality, can negatively impact blood sugar regulation and increase the risk of insulin resistance and type 2 diabetes.

To prioritize quality sleep and support blood sugar management, consider implementing the following sleep hygiene practices:

Consistent sleep schedule: To regulate your body's internal clock, go to bed and wake up at the same time every day, even on a weekend.
Create a Relaxing Bedtime Routine: Establish a calming bedtime routine to signal to your body that it's time to wind down and prepare for sleep. You can have a warm bath and do some relaxation techniques.

Optimize Your Sleep Environment: Create a comfortable sleep environment that is dark, quiet, and cool, with a supportive mattress and pillows.
Limit Screen Time Before Bed: Avoid electronic devices, such as smartphones, tablets, and computers, before bedtime, as the blue light emitted

from screens can interfere with melatonin production and disrupt sleep.

By prioritizing quality sleep and implementing healthy sleep habits, you can support blood sugar management and overall health and well-being.

In conclusion, lifestyle strategies such as regular exercise and physical activity, stress management techniques, and quality sleep play integral roles in blood sugar management. By incorporating these lifestyle interventions into your daily routine, you can optimize blood sugar levels, reduce the risk of insulin resistance and type 2 diabetes, and promote overall health and well-being. In the following chapters, we'll explore additional strategies for maintaining blood sugar balance through diet, medication, and other interventions.

CHAPTER SIX: SUPPLEMENTING YOUR DIET FOR BLOOD SUGAR SUPPORT

In this chapter, we'll explore various supplements and natural therapies that may support blood sugar regulation and promote overall health and well-being. While it's important to prioritize a balanced diet and lifestyle interventions, supplements and herbal remedies can complement these efforts and provide additional support for blood sugar management.

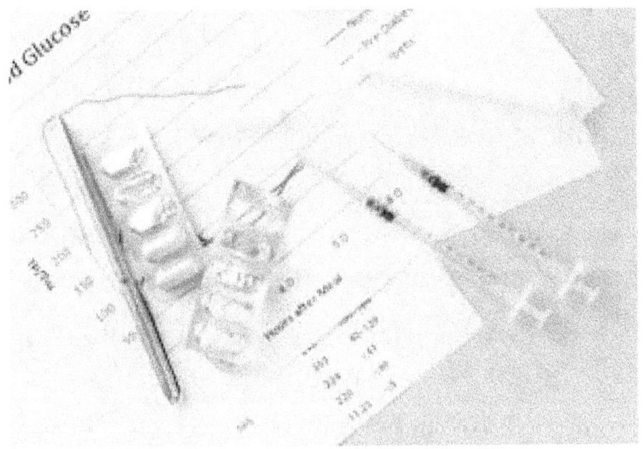

Essential Nutrients for Blood Sugar Health

Several nutrients play important roles in blood sugar regulation and insulin sensitivity. Including these nutrients in your diet can help support optimal blood sugar levels and overall metabolic health:

Chromium: Chromium is a mineral that enhances insulin sensitivity and helps regulate blood sugar levels. Good food sources of chromium include broccoli, nuts, whole grains, and brewer's yeast.

Magnesium: Magnesium is involved in glucose metabolism and insulin action. Consuming magnesium-rich foods such as leafy green vegetables, nuts, seeds, and whole grains can support blood sugar health.

Omega-3 Fatty Acids: Omega-3 fatty acids have anti-inflammatory properties and may improve insulin sensitivity. Excellent sources of omega-3s are fatty fish such as salmon, mackerel, and sardines.

Vitamin D: Vitamin D deficiency has been linked to insulin resistance and type 2 diabetes. Sun exposure and dietary sources such as fatty fish, fortified dairy products, and egg yolks can help maintain adequate vitamin D levels.

Including these essential nutrients in your diet through whole foods is the best way to ensure optimal blood sugar health. However, if you're unable to meet your nutrient needs through diet alone, supplements may be considered.

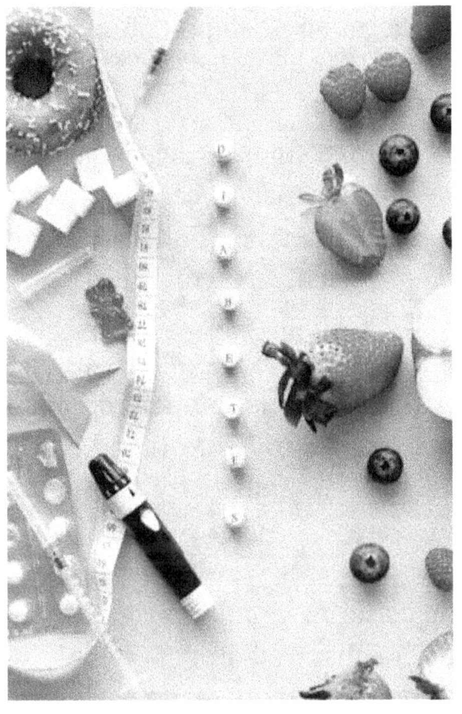

Supplements for Blood Sugar Regulation

Several supplements have been studied for their potential benefits in supporting blood sugar regulation. While more research is needed to confirm their effectiveness, some supplements that may offer blood sugar support include:

Alpha-Lipoic Acid: Alpha-lipoic acid is an antioxidant that may improve insulin sensitivity and reduce oxidative stress. It can be found in small amounts in foods like spinach, broccoli, and yeast, but supplements are also available.
 Berberine: Several plants, including goldenseal and barberry, are known to contain a compound called Berberino. It has been shown to lower blood sugar levels and improve insulin sensitivity in some studies.

Cinnamon: Cinnamon contains compounds that may mimic the effects of insulin and improve glucose uptake by cells. Adding cinnamon to your diet or taking cinnamon supplements may help support blood sugar regulation.

Fiber Supplements: Soluble fiber supplements such as psyllium husk or glucomannan can help slow down the absorption of carbohydrates and promote stable blood sugar levels.

Before taking any supplements for blood sugar regulation, it's important to consult with a healthcare professional, as some supplements may interact with medications or have side effects.

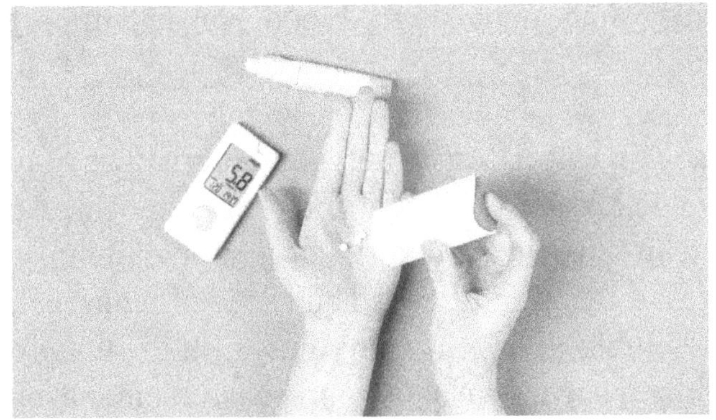

Herbal Remedies and Natural Therapies

In addition to supplements, several herbal remedies and natural therapies have been used traditionally to support blood sugar management. Some herbs and botanicals that may offer blood sugar support include:

Ginseng: Ginseng is an adaptogenic herb that may improve insulin sensitivity and enhance glucose metabolism. You can take it as a supplement, or drink it like tea. Fenugreek: The seeds of fenugreek contain soluble fiber and compounds that may help reduce blood sugar levels. Fenugreek supplements or tea may be beneficial for blood sugar regulation.

Bitter Melon: Bitter melon contains compounds that may mimic the effects of insulin and improve glucose uptake by cells. It is commonly used in traditional medicine for blood sugar management.
While herbal remedies and natural therapies can complement dietary and lifestyle interventions for blood sugar management, it's important to use them under the guidance of a healthcare professional, especially if you are on medications.

In conclusion, supplementing your diet with essential nutrients, supplements, herbal remedies, and natural therapies may provide additional support for blood sugar regulation and overall metabolic health. While these interventions can be beneficial, they should not replace a balanced diet and healthy lifestyle habits. Before starting any supplements or herbal remedies, consult with a healthcare professional to ensure they are safe and appropriate for your individual needs. In the following chapters, we'll explore additional strategies for maintaining blood sugar balance through lifestyle modifications and medication, when necessary.

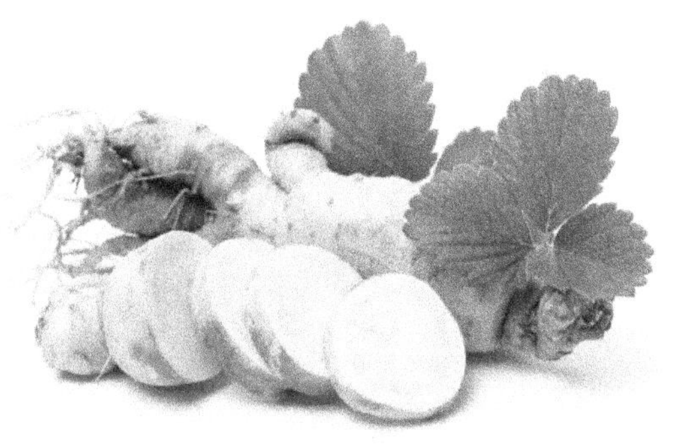

CHAPTER SEVEN: MONITORING AND ADJUSTING YOUR PLAN

In this chapter, we'll discuss the importance of monitoring your blood sugar levels, identifying signs of imbalance, and making adjustments to your diet and lifestyle plan for optimal blood sugar management and overall health.

Tracking Progress: Keeping a Blood Sugar Journal Keeping a blood sugar journal is a valuable tool for monitoring your progress and identifying patterns in your blood sugar levels over time. By recording your blood sugar readings, meals, physical activity, medication, and other relevant factors, you can gain valuable insights into how various factors affect your blood sugar levels.

When keeping a blood sugar journal, be sure to include the following information:

Blood Sugar Readings: Record your blood sugar levels at different times of the day, such as before and after meals, before bedtime, and during periods of physical activity or stress.

Meals and Snacks: Note the types and amounts of foods and beverages you consume, as well as the timing of your meals and snacks.

Physical Activity: Record the duration and intensity of your exercise and physical activity, as well as any changes in your blood sugar levels before and after activity.

Medication and Supplements: Keep track of any medications, supplements, or herbal remedies you're taking, as well as the dosage and timing.
By regularly reviewing your blood sugar journal, you can identify trends, triggers, and areas for improvement in your blood sugar management plan.

Identifying Signs of Imbalance

It's essential to be aware of the signs and symptoms of blood sugar imbalance, as well as the factors that can affect blood sugar levels. Common signs of low blood sugar (hypoglycemia) include:

Shakiness
Sweating
Dizziness
Confusion
Hunger
Rapid heartbeat
Irritability
On the other hand, high blood sugar (hyperglycemia) may present with symptoms such as:

Increased thirst
Frequent urination
Fatigue
Blurred vision
Slow wound healing
Recurrent infections
If you experience any of these symptoms, it's important to check your blood sugar levels and take appropriate action to address the imbalance.

Making Adjustments for Optimal Health

Based on the information gathered from your blood sugar journal and your awareness of signs of imbalance, you can make adjustments to your diet, physical activity, medication, and lifestyle habits to optimize your blood sugar management plan.

Some adjustments you may consider include:

Diet Modifications: Adjust your carbohydrate intake, meal timing, and portion sizes to better control blood sugar levels. Experiment with different foods and meal combinations to see how they affect your blood sugar.

Physical Activity: Increase or modify your exercise routine to better regulate blood sugar levels. Take your routine to a whole new level by incorporating aerobics, strength training, and flexibility exercises.

Medication Management: Work with your healthcare provider to adjust your medication regimen as needed based on your blood sugar readings and overall health status.

Lifestyle Changes: Implement stress management techniques, prioritize quality sleep, and address any other lifestyle factors that may impact blood sugar levels.

By making regular adjustments to your blood sugar management plan based on ongoing monitoring and evaluation, you can optimize your health and well-being.

In conclusion, monitoring your blood sugar levels, identifying signs of imbalance, and making appropriate adjustments to your diet, physical activity, medication, and lifestyle habits are essential for optimal blood sugar management and overall health. By keeping a blood sugar journal, staying vigilant for signs of imbalance, and being proactive about making adjustments as needed, you can take control of your blood sugar levels and live a healthier, more vibrant life. In the following chapters, we'll explore additional strategies for maintaining blood sugar balance through lifestyle modifications, medication, and other interventions.

CHAPTER EIGHT: OVERCOMING CHALLENGES AND STAYING MOTIVATED

In this chapter, we'll discuss strategies for overcoming common challenges faced when managing blood sugar levels and staying motivated on your journey to better health. From dealing with cravings and temptations to navigating social situations and dining out, as well as maintaining a positive mindset and staying focused on your goals, you'll learn practical tips for overcoming obstacles and staying on track with your blood sugar management plan.

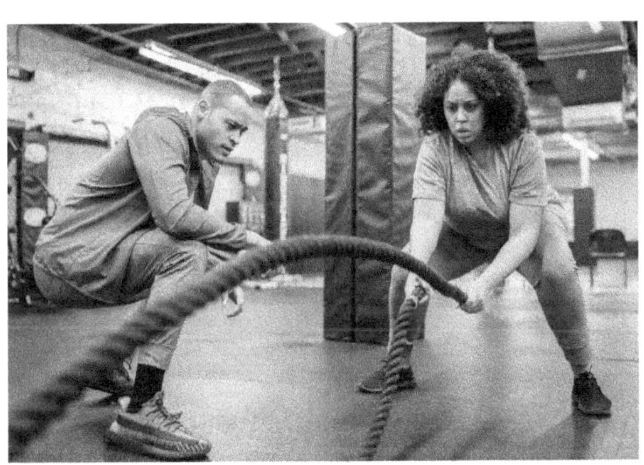

Dealing with Cravings and Temptations

Cravings and temptations for high-carbohydrate, sugary foods can be challenging to resist, especially when trying to manage blood sugar levels. However, there are several strategies you can employ to help manage cravings and stay on track with your dietary goals:

Plan for the future: Prepare healthy snacks and meals in advance to have on hand when cravings arise. Choose nutrient-dense options that satisfy your hunger and cravings without causing blood sugar spikes.

Practice Portion Control: Allow yourself to enjoy small portions of your favorite treats occasionally, but be mindful of portion sizes and their impact on blood sugar levels.

Find Healthier Alternatives: Look for healthier alternatives to your favorite high-carb or sugary foods. For example, swap out sugary snacks for fresh fruit, or opt for whole-grain alternatives to refined carbohydrates.

Stay hydrated: If thirst is sometimes mistaken for hunger, drink plenty of water throughout the day. Staying hydrated can help curb cravings and keep you feeling satisfied.

By being mindful of your cravings, planning, and making healthier choices, you can better manage cravings and maintain control over your blood sugar levels.

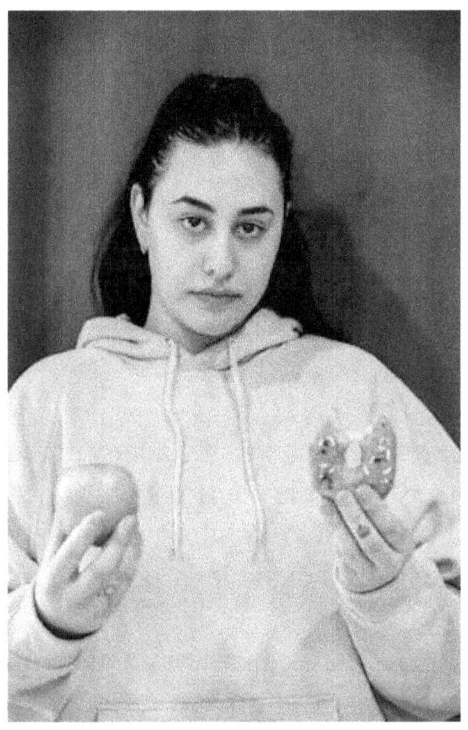

Handling Social Situations and Dining Out

Social situations and dining out can present unique challenges when managing blood sugar levels, but with some planning and preparation, you can navigate these situations successfully:

Communicate Your Needs: Don't be afraid to communicate your dietary preferences and needs to friends, family, and restaurant staff. Many restaurants are willing to accommodate special requests and dietary restrictions.

Preview Menus: Before dining out, take a look at the menu online to identify healthier options that align with your dietary goals. Look for dishes that are lower in carbohydrates and include lean protein and non-starchy vegetables.

Be Mindful of Portions: Pay attention to portion sizes when dining out, as restaurant portions are often larger than what you would typically eat at home. Consider splitting a meal with a dining companion or asking for a half portion.

Make Smart Substitutions: When ordering, ask for substitutions or modifications to make your meal healthier. For example, request steamed vegetables instead of fries or a side salad instead of bread.

By planning, communicating your needs, and making smart choices when dining out, you can enjoy social occasions while still maintaining control over your blood sugar levels.

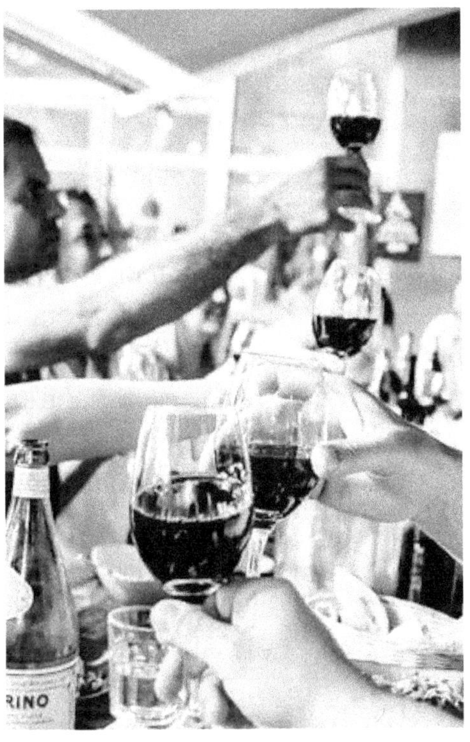

Staying Positive and Focused on Your Goals

Maintaining a positive mindset and staying focused on your goals are essential for long-term success in managing blood sugar levels:

Set realistic targets: set achievable benchmarks for yourself and celebrate how far you've come. To keep you motivated, break bigger goals into smaller, more manageable steps. Stay Connected: Surround yourself with a supportive network of friends, family, or a healthcare team who can provide accountability and encouragement. Share your successes and challenges with others who understand and can offer support.

Practice Self Compassion: Be kind to yourself, and realize that setbacks are a normal part of the journey. Instead of dwelling on mistakes, focus on what you can learn from them and how you can move forward.

Celebrate Your Successes: Celebrate your accomplishments, no matter how small. Whether it's reaching a blood sugar milestone, sticking to your meal plan for the day, or incorporating more physical activity into your routine, take time to acknowledge and celebrate your achievements.

By staying positive, setting realistic goals, and maintaining focus on your long-term health and well-being, you can overcome challenges and stay motivated on your journey to better blood sugar management.

Lastly, overcoming challenges and staying motivated when managing blood sugar levels requires planning, preparation, and a positive mindset. By implementing strategies for dealing with cravings and temptations, navigating social situations and dining out, and maintaining focus on your goals, you can successfully manage blood sugar levels and achieve better health and well-being. In the following chapters, we'll explore additional tips and strategies for maintaining blood sugar balance and living a healthier, more vibrant life.

CHAPTER NINE:
ADDITIONAL STRATEGIES FOR
BLOOD SUGAR MANAGEMENT

In this chapter, we'll delve deeper into additional strategies for managing blood sugar levels and promoting overall health and well-being. From incorporating specific dietary approaches to exploring the role of stress management and mindfulness practices, as well as discussing the potential benefits of complementary therapies, you'll discover a comprehensive range of tools and techniques for optimizing blood sugar health.

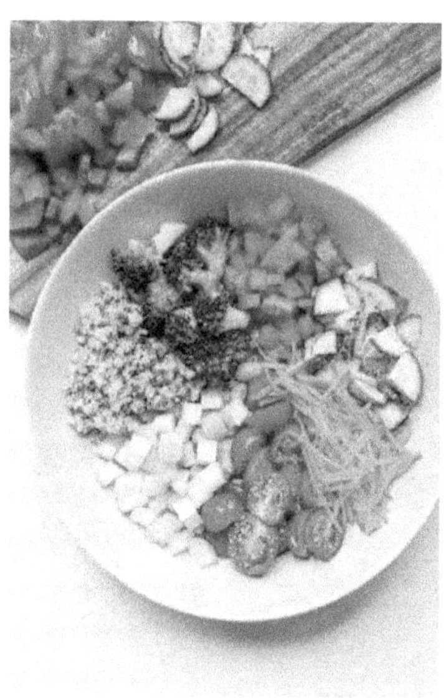

Dietary Approaches for Blood Sugar Management

While we've discussed the importance of balanced meals and smart food choices in previous chapters, there are specific dietary approaches that may offer additional benefits for managing blood sugar levels:

Low-Carb Diet: Some research suggests that reducing carbohydrate intake, particularly refined carbohydrates and sugars, can help stabilize blood sugar levels and improve insulin sensitivity. A low-carb diet focuses on minimizing the consumption of foods high in carbohydrates and prioritizing protein, healthy fats, and non-starchy vegetables.

Intermittent Fasting: Intermittent fasting involves alternating periods of eating and fasting, which may help regulate blood sugar levels and improve metabolic health. By limiting the window of time in which you consume food, intermittent fasting can help reduce insulin resistance and promote fat burning.

Plant-based diet: whole, minimally processed plant foods such as fruits, vegetables, whole grains, legumes, nuts, and seeds are the focus of a plant-based diet. Research suggests that a plant-based diet rich in fiber, antioxidants, and phytonutrients can help improve insulin sensitivity, reduce inflammation, and support overall health.

By exploring these dietary approaches and experimenting with different meal plans and eating patterns, you can find what works best for you and your blood sugar health.

Stress Management and Mindfulness Practices

Chronic stress can have a significant impact on blood sugar levels and overall health, so it's essential to incorporate stress management and mindfulness practices into your daily routine:

Mindful Eating: Practice mindful eating by paying attention to the sensory experience of eating, including the taste, texture, and aroma of food. Mindful eating can help you become more attuned to your body's hunger and fullness cues and prevent overeating.

Breathing Exercises: Engage in deep breathing exercises to promote relaxation and reduce stress levels. Take slow, deep breaths, focusing on the rise and fall of your abdomen with each inhale and exhale. Deep breathing can activate the body's relaxation response and counteract the effects of stress on blood sugar levels.

Mindfulness Meditation: Dedicate time each day to mindfulness meditation practice, focusing on your breath, sensations in your body, or sounds in your environment. Mindfulness meditation can help reduce stress, improve emotional well-being, and enhance self-awareness.

By incorporating stress management and mindfulness practices into your daily routine, you can reduce the impact of stress on blood sugar levels and promote overall health and well-being.

Complementary Therapies for Blood Sugar Health
In addition to dietary and lifestyle interventions, some complementary therapies may offer benefits for managing blood sugar levels and supporting overall health:

Acupuncture: Acupuncture is an ancient healing technique from China that involves the insertion of small needles in specific parts of the body to boost energy flow and increase recovery. In some studies, acupuncture has been shown to enhance insulin sensitivity and decrease blood sugar levels in diabetic patients.
Yoga: Research indicates that yoga may help improve blood sugar control, reduce insulin resistance, and enhance overall well-being in individuals with diabetes.
Herbal Remedies: Certain herbs and botanicals have been used traditionally to support blood sugar regulation. For example, bitter melon, fenugreek, and cinnamon are herbs that may help lower blood sugar levels and improve insulin sensitivity. While more research is needed to confirm their effectiveness, some people find herbal remedies helpful as part of their blood sugar management plan.

Before incorporating complementary therapies into your blood sugar management plan, it's essential to consult with a healthcare professional to ensure they are safe and appropriate for your individual needs.

Summary and Conclusion
In conclusion, managing blood sugar levels requires a multifaceted approach that addresses dietary, lifestyle, and emotional factors. By incorporating specific dietary approaches, such as low-carb, intermittent fasting, or plant-based diets, and exploring stress management and mindfulness practices, you can optimize blood sugar health and promote overall well-being. Additionally, complementary therapies like acupuncture, yoga, and herbal remedies may offer additional support for managing blood sugar levels and enhancing metabolic health.

As you continue your journey to better blood sugar health, remember to stay curious, stay proactive, and stay committed to your well-being. Experiment with different strategies, listen to your body and seek support from healthcare professionals and loved ones as needed. With dedication, perseverance, and a holistic approach to health, you can achieve better blood sugar control and live a healthier life.

CHAPTER TEN:
TAKING ACTION: PRACTICAL STEPS FOR MANAGING YOUR BLOOD SUGAR LEVELS

In this final chapter, we'll explore practical steps you can take to effectively manage your blood sugar levels and promote overall health and well-being. From monitoring your blood sugar levels to making informed food choices and incorporating regular physical activity, you'll discover actionable strategies to help you take control of your blood sugar health.

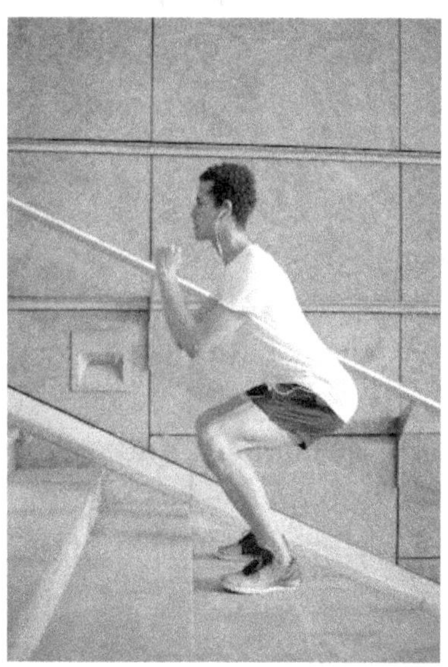

Monitoring Your Blood Sugar Levels

Regular monitoring of your blood sugar levels is essential for understanding how your body responds to different foods, activities, and lifestyle habits. Here are some practical steps for monitoring your blood sugar levels effectively:

Use a Glucose Meter: Invest in a reliable glucose meter and test strips to monitor your blood sugar levels at home. Follow the manufacturer's instructions for accurate testing and record your readings in a logbook or smartphone app.

Establish Testing Routine: Develop a consistent testing routine by testing your blood sugar levels at the same times each day, such as before and after meals, before bedtime, and during periods of physical activity or stress.

Track Trends and Patterns: Review your blood sugar readings regularly to identify trends and patterns in your blood sugar levels. Look for factors that may influence your readings, such as meal timing, food choices, physical activity, and stress levels.

Share Results with Healthcare Provider: Share your blood sugar logbook or app data with your healthcare provider during regular check-ups. Your healthcare provider can help interpret your readings and make adjustments to your treatment plan as needed.

By monitoring your blood sugar levels regularly and tracking trends over time, you can gain valuable insights into how different factors impact your blood sugar health and make informed decisions to better manage your levels.

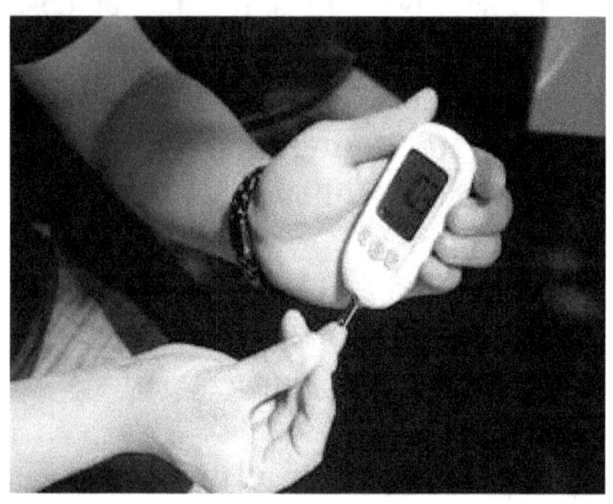

Making Informed Food Choices

Diet plays a crucial role in blood sugar management, so making informed food choices is key to maintaining stable blood sugar levels. To make healthy food choices, here are some practical tips:

Focus on whole foods: include whole, minimally processed foods in your diet, such as fruits, vegetables, whole grains, lean proteins, and healthy fats. These foods are rich in nutrients and fiber, which can help regulate blood sugar levels.

Limit Added Sugars and Refined Carbohydrates: Reduce your intake of foods and beverages high in added sugars and refined carbohydrates, such as sugary drinks, sweets, pastries, and white bread. These foods can cause blood sugar spikes and contribute to insulin resistance over time.

Choose Carbohydrates Appropriately: choose simple carbohydrates with a low Glycemic Index, e.g. grains, legumes, and non-starchy vegetables. These carbohydrates are absorbed more slowly, which results in increased blood sugar levels over time.

Practice Portion Control: Be mindful of portion sizes and avoid oversized servings, especially high-carb foods. Use smaller plates and bowls, and listen to your body's hunger and fullness cues to avoid overeating.

Balance Your Plate: Aim to create balanced meals that include a mix of carbohydrates, protein, and healthy fats. This combination can help stabilize blood sugar levels and promote satiety.

By making informed food choices and prioritizing whole, nutrient-dense foods in your diet, you can better regulate your blood sugar levels and support overall health and well-being.

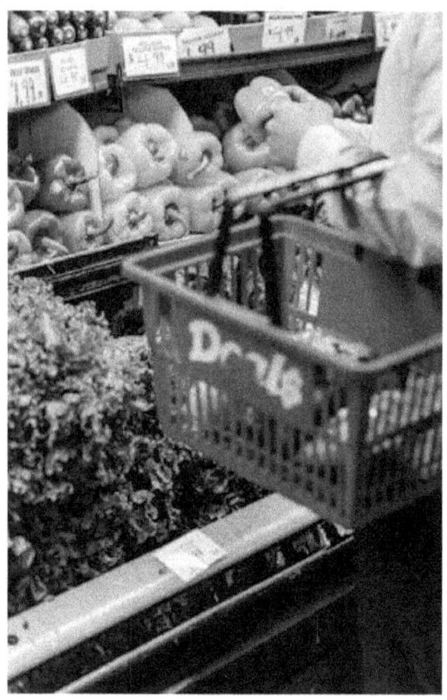

Incorporating Regular Physical Activity

Physical activity is another essential component of blood sugar management, as it helps improve insulin sensitivity and glucose uptake by cells. Here are some practical ways to incorporate regular physical activity into your routine:

Find Activities You Enjoy: Choose physical activities that you enjoy and look forward to, whether it's walking, cycling, swimming, dancing, or gardening. Finding activities that are enjoyable and sustainable for you is the key. Set realistic goals: Set realistic goals for physical activity and gradually increase the intensity and duration of your exercise. Get started with small, attainable goals and celebrate your progress in this journey.

Make It Social: Exercise with friends, family, or a workout buddy to stay motivated and accountable. Join a fitness class, sports team, or walking group to make physical activity more social and enjoyable.
Incorporate Movement Into Your Day: Look for opportunities to incorporate movement into your daily routine, such as taking the stairs instead of the elevator, walking or biking to work, or doing household chores like gardening or cleaning.
Be Consistent: Aim for at least 150 minutes of moderate-intensity aerobic exercise or 75 minutes of

vigorous-intensity aerobic exercise per week, along with two or more days of strength training exercises targeting major muscle groups.

By incorporating regular physical activity into your routine, you can improve your overall fitness, enhance insulin sensitivity, and better regulate your blood sugar levels.

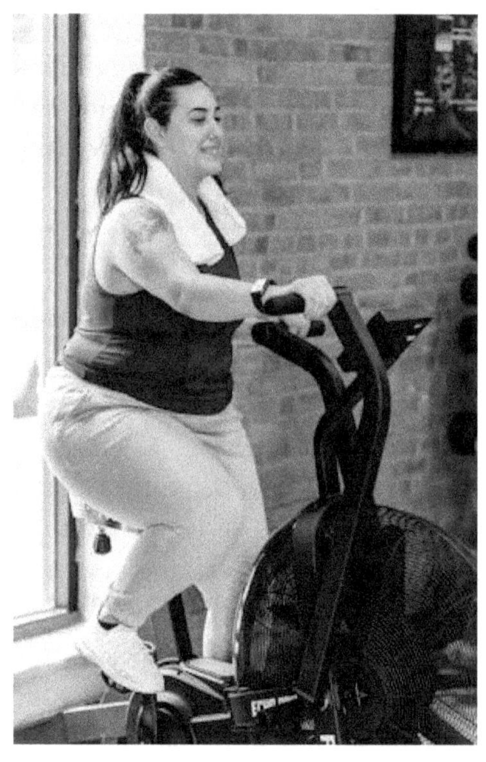

CONCLUSION

As we conclude our journey together through the pages of this book, it's essential to reflect on the progress we've made, celebrate our successes, and look ahead to the future with optimism and determination. Throughout this exploration of managing blood sugar health, we've uncovered a wealth of knowledge and practical strategies to support our well-being and vitality.

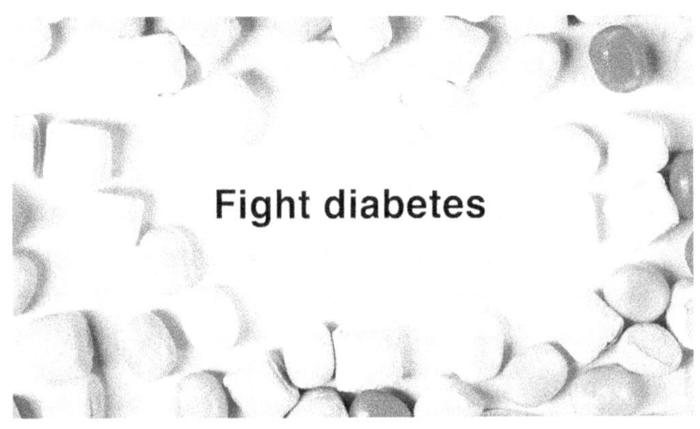

Celebrating Your Successes

First and foremost, I want to extend my heartfelt congratulations to you for embarking on this journey to better blood sugar health. Each step you've taken, each positive change you've made, is a testament to your dedication and commitment to your well-being. Whether you've made significant lifestyle adjustments or small, incremental changes, every effort you've made is worthy of celebration.

Take a moment to acknowledge and celebrate your successes, no matter how big or small they may seem. Celebrate the times you chose a nourishing meal over a sugary snack, the moments you prioritized self-care and stress management, and the milestones you've reached on your journey to better blood sugar health. By recognizing and celebrating your successes, you reinforce positive habits and build momentum for continued progress.

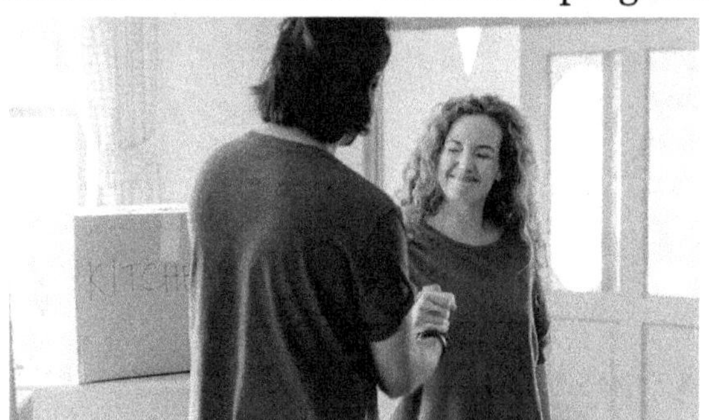

Continuing Your Journey to Better Blood Sugar Health

While this book may be coming to a close, your journey to better blood sugar health is far from over. It's just the beginning. As you move forward, I encourage you to continue exploring and experimenting with the strategies and techniques you've learned here. Your journey is unique, and what works best for you may differ from what works for others.

Continue to prioritize balanced meals, regular physical activity, stress management, and mindfulness practices in your daily routine. Stay curious and open-minded, and be willing to adapt and adjust your approach as needed. Pay attention to how your body responds to different foods, activities, and lifestyle habits, and make choices that align with your individual needs and preferences.

Remember that progress is not always linear. There may be setbacks along the way, but each setback presents an opportunity for growth and learning. Approach challenges with resilience and determination, and don't be afraid to ask for support from healthcare professionals, loved ones, and community resources when needed.

As you continue your journey to better blood sugar health, keep these key principles in mind:

Consistency: Stay consistent with your healthy habits, even on days when motivation is low or obstacles arise. Small, consistent actions over time can lead to significant improvements in blood sugar control and overall well-being.

Self-Compassion: Be kind to yourself and practice self-compassion as you navigate challenges and setbacks. Remember that you are human, and it's okay to make mistakes. Treat yourself with the same kindness and understanding you would offer to a friend facing similar struggles.

Curiosity: Maintain a sense of curiosity and exploration as you discover what works best for you. Stay open to trying new foods, activities, and approaches to managing blood sugar levels, and be willing to adjust your plan based on feedback from your body.

Empowerment: Recognize the power you have to take control of your health and well-being. You are the author of your health journey, and your choices and actions have the potential to shape your future in profound ways.

Continuing your journey to better blood sugar health requires dedication and persistence. Stay consistent with monitoring your blood sugar levels, making informed food choices, and incorporating regular physical activity into your routine. Educate yourself about blood sugar health, seek support from healthcare professionals and loved ones, and celebrate your progress along the way. Set realistic goals, prioritize self-care, and maintain a positive mindset as you navigate the ups and downs of managing your blood sugar levels. Remember, every positive choice you make brings you one step closer to achieving better blood sugar control.

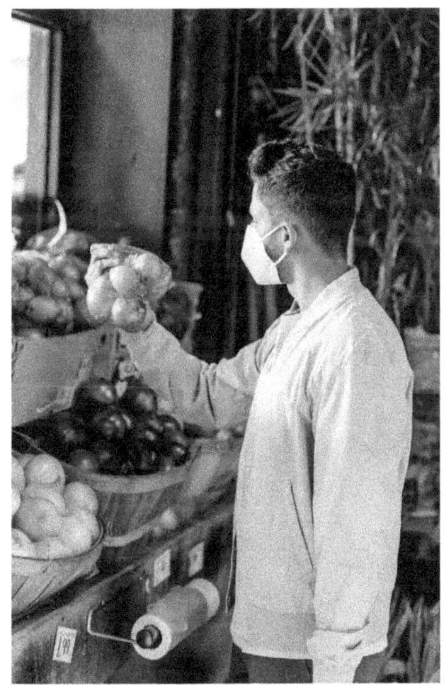

In conclusion, as we bid farewell to this journey through the world of blood sugar health, I want to express my gratitude for allowing me to be a part of your path to wellness. It has been an honor and a privilege to share this knowledge and experience with you, and I hope you feel empowered and inspired to continue your journey to better blood sugar health.

Remember that you are capable, you are resilient, and you are deserving of vibrant health and vitality. Keep moving forward with courage and determination, and never lose sight of the incredible potential that lies within you.